KT-226-022

It's Your Health!

Eating Properly

JONATHAN REES

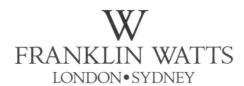

FRANKLIN WATTS
LONDON • SYDNEY

First published in 2004 by Franklin Watts
338 Euston Road
London NW1 3BH

Franklin Watts Australia
Hachette Children's Books
Level 17/207 Kent Street
Sydney NSW 2000

Series editor: Sarah Peutrill
Editor: Sarah Ridley
Designer: Reg Cox, Pewter Design
Series design: Peter Scoulding
Illustration: Mike Atkinson and Guy Smith, Mainline Design, and James Evans
Picture researcher: Sophie Hartley
Series consultant: Wendy Anthony, Health Education Unit, Education Service, Birmingham City Council
Picture credits: Photo from www.JohnBirdsall.co.uk: 26. BSIP, Laurent/Science Photo Library: 19b. © Phillip Carr/Photofusion: 9tl. Digital Vision Ltd.: 13, 34. Chris Fairclough/Franklin Watts: 11, 23, 27b, 29b. Franklin Watts: 4, 12, 18, 19t, 21, 22, 32, 33t, 37b, 39t, 45. © Gina Glover/Photofusion: 41b. © Jaume Gual/Powerstock: 41t. David Hoffman Photo Library/Alamy: 35b. © Reed Kaestner/Corbis: 17b. © Michael Kim/Corbis: 29t. Art Kowalsky/Alamy: 40. Andy Levin/Science Photo Library: 8.© C. Macpherson/Photofusion: 24. Andrew McClenaghan/Science Photo Library: 27t. Ray Moller/Franklin Watts: 9tr & b, 14, 15, 16, 17t, 20, 38. © Robert Morris/Photofusion: 35t. © Anthony Sanger-Davies/Photofusion: 37t. Jane Shemilt/Science Photo Library: 33b. © Emma Smith/Photofusion: 28. Sheila Terry/Science Photo Library: 30, 31b. Mark Thomas/Science Photo Library: 31t. Topham Picturepoint: 36. © Michael S. Yamashita/Corbis: 39b. Every attempt has been made to clear copyright. Should there be any inadvertent omission, please apply to the publisher for rectification.

The Publisher would like to thank the Brunswick Club for Young People, Fulham, London for their help with this book and our models.

A CIP catalogue record for this book is available from the British Library

ISBN: 978 0 7496 5571 6

Printed in Malaysia

Franklin Watts is a division of Hachette Children's Books.

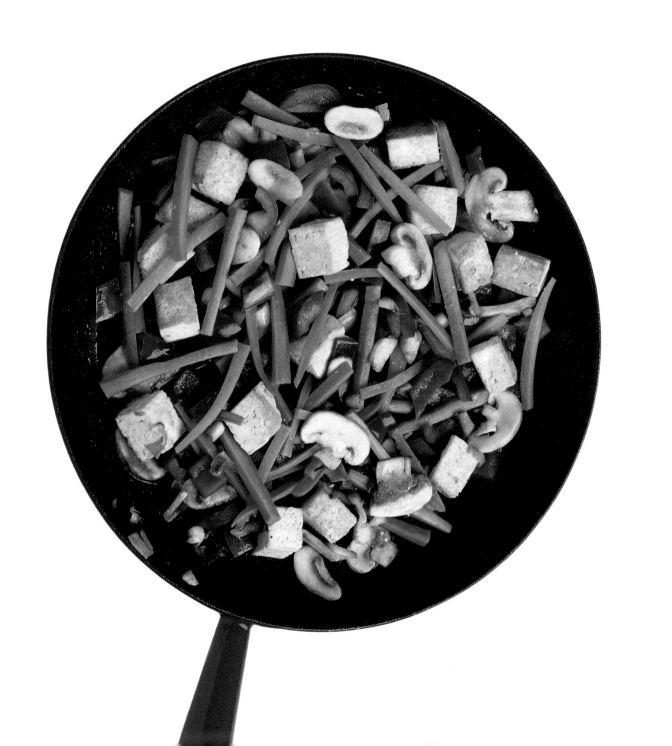

Contents

Why do we need food?

All animals have to eat to survive, and humans are no different. Food is essential because it supplies our bodies with the energy we use for living and being active. Eating the right food keeps us healthy and helps to protect our bodies from disease. But eating should be so much more than this – an enjoyable experience, a celebration or a way of relaxing with our families and friends.

It's your decision

Do you think about where your food comes from?
Whether it arrives by road or air, it will have contributed to atmospheric pollution. How was the food grown? Some people prefer to buy 'fair trade' food, because they think farmers in developing countries get a better deal this way.

Nutrients

When we eat, our bodies use the parts of the food called nutrients to run our body functions. The nutrients we need include carbohydrates, proteins and fats, as well as vitamins and minerals. Both fats and carbohydrates provide us with most of the energy we use. Proteins are used to help our body cells grow and repair themselves.

The nation's diet

What people eat varies around the world. A nation's traditional diet is based on what can be grown easily in that country. So, people who live in India and China eat a diet based on rice, with vegetables and some protein – meat, fish or pulses. People living in cooler climates tend to eat a more wheat-based diet with bread or pasta to accompany meat, fish and vegetables.

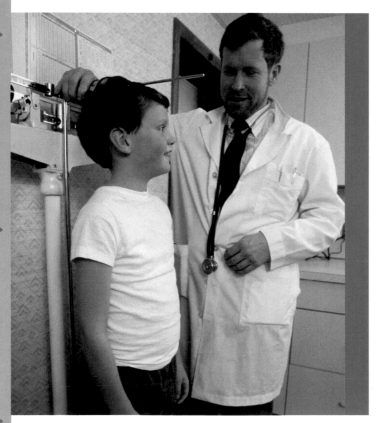

Nutrients such as proteins help us to grow.

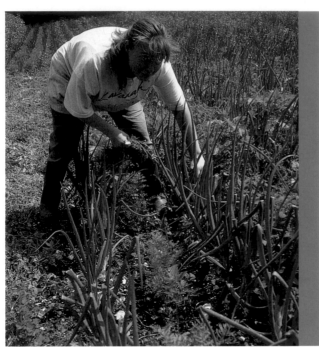

It's your experience

'I like all sorts of food, but for me there's nothing more delicious than the food my mum and me grow in our garden. It's fresh, tasty and, best of all, it's free!'

Jez, aged 15

People who are able to grow their own food benefit from the freshest foods straight to the table!

What we need	Found in
Carbohydrates	Starchy foods like bread, potatoes and pasta, as well as in sweet foods like cakes and biscuits.
Proteins	Foods like meat, fish, dairy products, pulses and nuts.
Fats	Foods like butter and vegetable oil, as well as meat, fish and nuts.
Vitamins and minerals	Many foods. Meat, fish, pulses and green vegetables contain iron that helps our blood to carry oxygen around the body. Oranges and many fruits are a good source of vitamin C, a chemical that protects our bodies against illnesses and infections and helps absorb iron. Other vitamins occur in a wide range of vegetables and fruits (see pages 20-21).
Fibre	Many foods contain a substance called fibre, which is itself found in cereals like wheat, and fruit and vegetables. Fibre is not a nutrient as our bodies cannot absorb any goodness from it, but it adds bulk to many foods and is extremely helpful in keeping the digestive process moving.
Water	Our bodies need lots of water every day to keep us healthy. Water is one of the main ingredients in many foods but we also need to drink at least eight glasses of water per day.

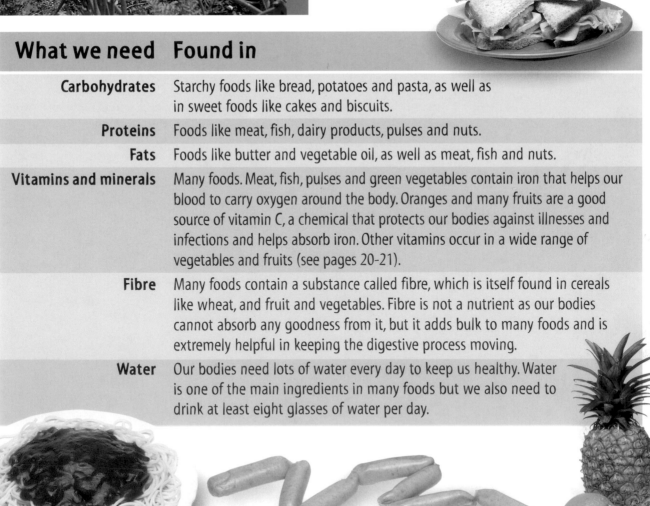

How our bodies break down food

When we eat, our bodies break down the food and absorb its nutrients. This is called digestion and it starts the moment we take the first bite of food.

It's your opinion

The digestive system is like a finely-balanced machine. What do you think you can do to keep it running as smoothly as possible?

The digestive system

Mouth

Throat

Oesophagus

Stomach

Small intestine

Rectum

Large intestine

Anus

1. Digestion starts in the mouth where we chew our food with our teeth. This breaks the food into smaller pieces so that the chemicals in our bodies can act more efficiently on it. Saliva is also added to the food at this point, to make the food softer and easier to swallow. It also starts breaking food down using chemicals called enzymes.

2. Food passes down the throat and oesophagus to the stomach where it is churned around a bit like clothes in a washing machine. Here more enzymes and a strong acid are added to the food, continuing the process of digestion.

3. From the stomach the food passes to the small intestine, a long coiled-up tube, where yet more enzymes are added. At this point some of the food has been broken down into particles called molecules. These nutrient molecules are small enough to be absorbed into the bloodstream.

4. The food that has not been absorbed then passes through another long tube called the large intestine where minerals and water are removed and faeces are formed. Faeces are all the leftovers that cannot easily be digested.

5. Faeces are then stored in the rectum until they are passed through the anus when we go to the toilet.

Our teeth are a very important part of the digestion process. We have different kinds of teeth to do different jobs when we eat food. We need to keep our teeth clean and healthy to eat properly.

Incisors (cut food)

Canines (grip and tear food)

Pre-molars (crush and chew food)

Molars (crush and chew food)

It's your experience

'Straight after school I feel exhausted. If I start eating biscuits, I can't stop so I often eat a sandwich or grab a banana to last me through to my evening meal. I soon feel more lively and can get on with my homework or talk to my friends.'

Kim, aged 13

How long does it take?

The whole process of digestion usually takes about 24-36 hours, but this does depend on how much we eat, how long we chew it and what it was that we ate. When the nutrients have been taken out of the food and are in the bloodstream, our bodies can then start to use them.

Some nutrients are used very quickly, supplying energy for many of the processes in our bodies, such as breathing, thinking and moving; others are used much more slowly, or even stored in body fat for future energy needs.

In the brain

The brain also takes part in the eating process. We do not have to remember to eat food. When our cells need food they send a signal to the brain. The brain then sends us a signal to tell us we are hungry.

The average person eats about 20 tonnes of food in their lifetime.

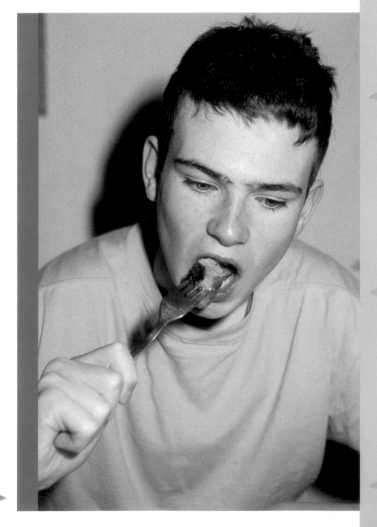

How much food do we need?

How much food a person needs depends on many things and varies from individual to individual. If someone leads a very busy life or if they do manual work, they will need to eat much more than a less active person. An athlete, for example, might need to eat food containing twice as much energy as an office-worker.

The same weight of food can contain vastly different amounts of calories or joules. The chart compares the number of calories in 100g of different food. The picture compares the number of calories in similar-sized portions of three types of food. ▼

The energy in our food

Energy is stored inside the food we eat. Each type of food contains different amounts of energy. Potatoes, rice, pasta and meat are full of energy and will supply us with energy for several hours. Eating a meal of just fruit or vegetables will not give the body as much energy so, although we may feel full temporarily, we will feel hungry again quite soon.

Measuring energy

The energy in food is measured in joules, with 1,000 joules written as 1kJ. Another measurement for energy is calories or kilocalories; 1Kcal is about the same as 4kJ. Although joules are the modern units that scientists use, most people still use calories to describe how much internal energy is in a food type.

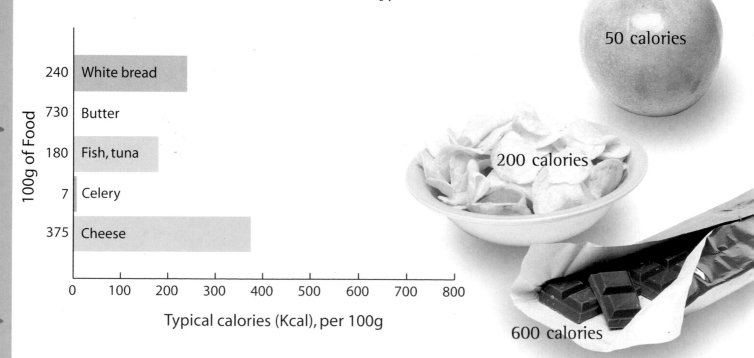

100g of Food

	Typical calories (Kcal), per 100g
240	White bread
730	Butter
180	Fish, tuna
7	Celery
375	Cheese

0   100   200   300   400   500   600   700   800

Typical calories (Kcal), per 100g

50 calories

200 calories

600 calories

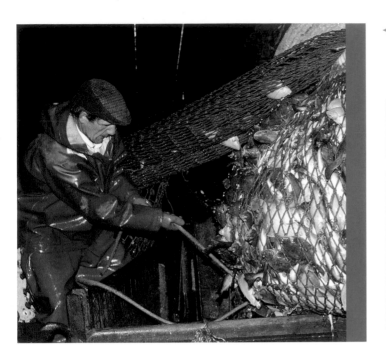

People who work in active jobs, like this fisherman, need to eat more calories to keep them going.

It's your experience

'My younger sister is really skinny; she easily eats as much as me and she doesn't do any exercise or anything but she never seems to put on weight. Dad says she's got a high metabolism and some people are just like that.'

Lilly, aged 15

Energy needs

Usually, the smaller someone is the less energy they need. So, children need less energy than adults. Women generally need less energy than men because men tend to be taller and have a greater proportion of muscle to fat in their bodies. Muscle cells use up more energy than fat cells.

Teenagers need more calories because their bodies are growing so rapidly, which requires a lot of energy.

Finally, some people need to eat more because they have very active lifestyles or because their bodies use energy faster than others. People who use energy faster have a high metabolic rate.

The wrong amount

One of the main reasons we eat food is because we get hungry. Hunger is the body's way of telling us we need to top up our energy supplies, a bit like the warning light in a car that reminds the driver to get more fuel.

However, if we ignore hunger signals and eat too little over the long term, we will lose weight. If we go without food completely we will eventually die.

On the other hand, if we eat more food than our bodies need, we do not use up all the energy. When this occurs, our bodies store the extra energy as fat, and we put on weight.

Average daily requirements

Person	Calories/Kcal
Inactive women/older adults	1,600
Children/inactive men/active women/ teenage girls	2,200
Active men/teenage boys	2,800

It's your opinion

People sometimes eat even though they are not hungry. What other reasons can you think of for why someone might want to eat?

Eating well

Most people in developed countries like western Europe and the USA get enough to eat. This has not always been the case and is still not true for many millions of people in the developing countries of the world. If we don't eat enough, not only will we be hungry, but we also risk being malnourished – when the body is not supplied with all the minerals, vitamins and everything else it needs to work properly.

Teenagers particularly need to pay attention to the amount of calcium they digest, as they are building up their adult skeleton which has to last for the rest of their lives. Lack of calcium caused by very low-fat diets at this important stage of development can lead to osteoporosis (weak bones) in later life.

A balanced diet

Food can be classified into different types as shown in the table on page 9. A healthy balanced diet should include a variety of different foods from each of the groups. This will give us plenty of the proteins, carbohydrates, fats, vitamins and minerals we need to grow and keep us feeling healthy.

Eating only certain food types, or not eating particular nutrients, can be very bad for us in the long run. If we eat a diet without enough proteins in it we may find that we become very tired or even that we do not grow normally. Avoiding carbohydrates denies our bodies the energy needed to function in the short and long term. Calcium, from vegetables and dairy products, is needed for healthy teeth and bones. Many people try not to eat too much fat as we know it isn't good for our health (see page 18), but we must eat some fats for our cells to work properly.

Recommendations

Some scientists and health officials are concerned about the types of food people eat. They know that many people eat too much fat and sugar and not enough fruit and vegetables, and that this leads to health problems (see pages 18-19). In the UK, Australia, Canada, New Zealand and some states in the USA the authorities are so concerned that they have advised everyone to eat at least five portions of fruit and vegetables each day (see pages 20-21). Many governments have also made official recommendations for how many of certain vitamins and minerals people should eat.

It's your experience

'My mum told me that I must eat at least five portions of fruit and vegetables every day, but I never do. I do have the odd apple sometimes but that's about it. I reckon she's talking rubbish – I'm perfectly healthy and I'm certainly not overweight.'

Josh, aged 13

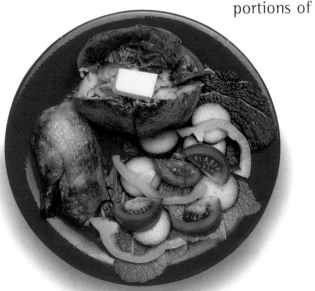

A balanced diet should include 30 per cent (maximum) of fats and sweets, 15 per cent of proteins, and 55 per cent of carbohydrates. This meal of a potato, chicken and salad is well-balanced.

It's your opinion

Most adults know so much about what they should and shouldn't eat. Why then do so many of them choose to ignore the advice? What do you think the government could do to help people eat better?

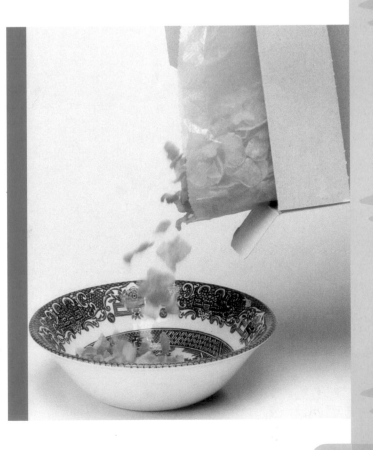

Most of us enjoy breakfast cereals in the morning or later in the day, as a quick snack. Many cereals are fortified with vitamins and minerals but it's best to choose the ones that are also low in salt and sugar.

Health-giving foods

Fresh fruit and vegetables are known to be vital for good health (see pages 20-21), but scientists have also discovered that certain other foods have properties that make them particularly good for us.

Oily fish such as trout is delicious and very good for us.

Fish

Oily fish such as tuna, mackerel, trout and salmon, are rich in omega-3 oils, oils that scientists have discovered are good for the brain, heart and joints. It is recommended that we all eat two portions of fish a week, including one portion of oily fish.

Milk

Milk has been considered a healthy food for many years. It is rich in protein, and also contains lots of calcium, a mineral that is essential for building strong and healthy bones and teeth.

Milk is very versatile and can be drunk on its own, poured on cereal or used in recipes.

Olive oil is a key ingredient in Mediterranean cooking.

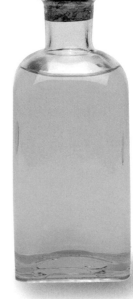

Cholesterol fighters

Other foods that people think may have health-giving properties include soya bean products, oats and olive oil, all of which may help reduce cholesterol levels in the bloodstream. There is also some evidence that red wine is good for you if drunk in moderation because it contains antioxidants – substances that can help fight several diseases.

Scientists are making new discoveries all the time about the properties of different foods. If you want to keep up-to-date you could look at one of the websites listed on page 43.

Add more fibre

Food that is high in fibre, such as wholemeal bread, beans and pulses, and many fruits and vegetables, is very good for our digestion. High-fibre and wholemeal foods have become very popular over the past few years as people have come to recognise the health benefits of eating them.

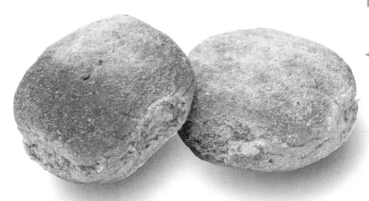

It's your experience

'I am fascinated by the ins and outs of what we are supposed to eat in a healthy diet. I particularly like it when I discover that something I enjoy eating, like salmon, is really good for me!'

Victoria , aged 18

Wholemeal bread is high in fibre. Fibre fill us up and helps to prevent constipation and some types of cancers.

Diets for long life

In southern Europe many people eat meals that include a lot of fish, olive oil and vegetables. This is called a Mediterranean diet and is thought to be one of the reasons that people in countries such as Italy and Greece can expect to live a long time. The Chinese and Japanese diets are also known to be very healthy; they are high in fish and contain lots of vegetables and soya bean products, like tofu.

It's your decision

Every day there seems to be a new bit of advice about what we should or shouldn't eat to keep us healthy. What simple changes could you make to your life so that you eat more healthily?

A Chinese family in Hong Kong enjoy a healthy meal.

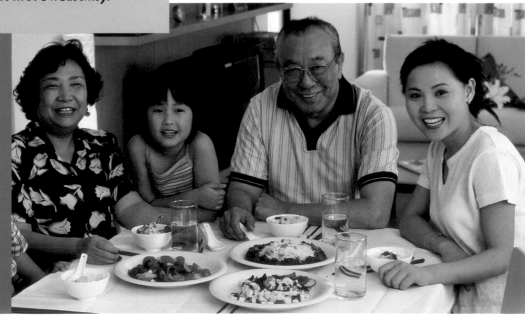

Problem foods

Just as some food is known to be good for our health, too much of some foods and drinks has quite the opposite effect. Sugar, salt and fat are an important part of everyone's diet, but eating too much of them will lead to health problems.

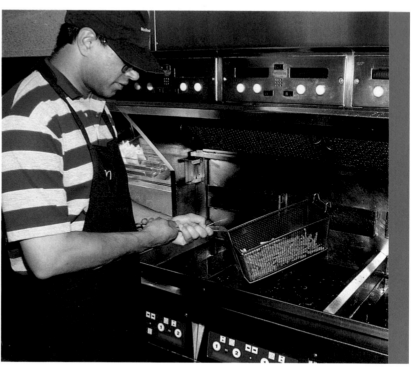

Fries absorb a lot of fat in the frying process. We should only eat them as an occasional treat.

Fat overload

Chips, cakes, chocolate bars, fried foods, dairy products and some meats are all high in fat. If we eat too much fatty food and don't burn it off with exercise or in our daily work, we will put on weight. If we become very over weight we are said to be obese, and this can be very bad for our health. In the UK and Australia, two in ten adults are obese, compared with one in ten in France. In the USA three in ten adults are classed as obese.

Salt

Eating too much salt can also result in high blood-pressure. The amount of salt we actually need to keep us healthy is about three grammes a day, which is about a quarter of what most people get.

Nutritionists advise that we should not add salt to our food in the cooking process or at the table. Salt is hidden in prepared meals, biscuits, bread and, more obviously, snack foods, such as crisps.

Heart disease

Heart disease kills over 150,000 people in the UK and over 500,000 in the USA each year. If we are very overweight our heart has to work harder to pump blood. Obesity can lead to high blood-pressure, which increases the risk of heart attacks by about 30 per cent and can cause a stroke.

Eating too many saturated fats, found in red meat, dairy products and many cakes and biscuits, increases levels of LDL (low-density lipoprotein), or 'bad cholesterol' in the blood. This can clog up arteries, preventing blood from reaching major organs and is a major cause of heart attacks.

It's your opinion

Most health problems take years to develop. Do you think you need to worry about your health and the food you eat now? When is the best time to consider what you eat and how it affects you?

It's your experience

'At school the other day we were learning about what makes a healthy diet. Then I got to the canteen and looked at what was on offer. What's the point of teaching us about good eating habits and then only offering chips and over-cooked vegetables, and cakes for pudding?'

Yasmin, aged 16

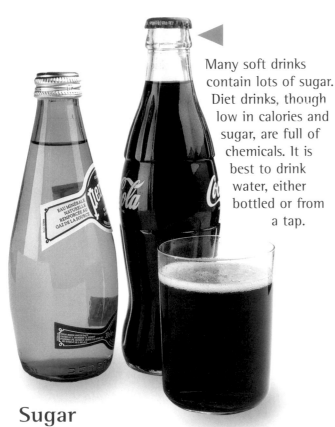

Many soft drinks contain lots of sugar. Diet drinks, though low in calories and sugar, are full of chemicals. It is best to drink water, either bottled or from a tap.

Sugar

Sugar is a kind of carbohydrate, but in a well-balanced diet most energy should come from starchy foods like bread and pasta. Sugar is found in syrup, treacle, jam, honey, raw cane sugar, glucose and fructose. We should cut down on sugar because, although it does give us a short burst of energy, it causes tooth decay and weight gain, as the excess sugar we don't use is converted into fat and stored.

Diabetes

Diabetes is a condition in which the body does not produce enough of the chemical insulin. Insulin controls how much sugar is in our bloodstream.

There are two types of diabetes. Type two is the most common type and is widespread in old people. Doctors are alarmed by the rise of type two diabetes in much younger people, even really young children. Research has shown that this is linked to the rising levels of obesity in young people. Scientists estimate that one in three Americans born in the year 2000 will develop the disease.

▼ Some diabetics have to inject themselves daily with artificial insulin.

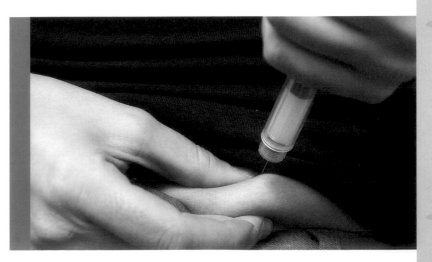

Five-a-day

Medical researchers continue to discover more about how to prevent certain life-threatening diseases, such as heart disease and some types of cancer. One 'wonder' food that keeps coming up in their research is the amazing benefit of eating a range of fresh fruit and vegetables.

Counting up the portions

We should all aim to eat at least five portions of fruit and vegetables (either fresh, tinned, frozen or dried) a day to supply us with all the vitamins and minerals we need. A portion is:

• Three heaped tablespoons of raw or cooked vegetables
• One apple, orange, pear or similar-sized fruit
• Two plums, tomatoes or similar-sized fruit
• One heaped tablespoon of dried fruit
• A dessert bowl of salad
• A glass of fruit juice (but juice can only count as one portion a day).

Changing your diet

Eating more fruit and vegetables doesn't mean that we have to give up our favourite foods. We just need to add much more fresh produce to what we are already eating. Try adding a banana to your cereal, a bowl of salad to your pasta supper, or reach for fruit as snacks between meals (for example, boxes of raisins are convenient to carry about in your bag). Use carrot or celery sticks with dips, rather than crisps, and add vegetables to your pizza.

▼ Which fruits and vegetables do you like to eat?

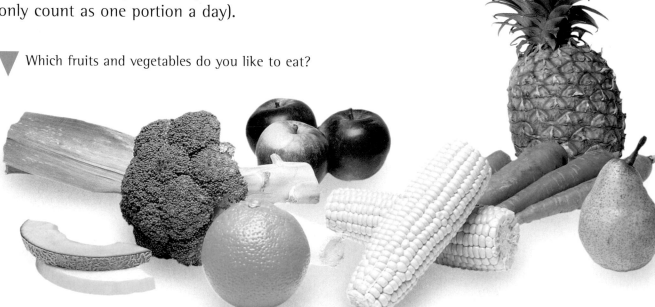

Health-giving properties

Scientific research has discovered that the colour of a particular fruit or vegetable is linked to some of its health-giving properties. Eating fruit and vegetables across the range of colours will ensure that your body receives everything it needs. The table shows just a few fruits and vegetables and some of their health-giving properties.

Although fruits and vegetables are full of beneficial natural vitamins, these can disappear as the food ages, or if the food is over-cooked.

Food	Contains	Good for
Tomatoes, strawberries and peppers	Lypocene gives the red colour, Vitamin C*	May reduce the risk of certain cancers
Peppers, oranges, lemons and carrots	Betacarotene gives the orange/yellow colour Vitamin C	Helps maintain good eyesight
Plums, blueberries and purple grapes	Anthocyanin, Vitamin C	Thought to have an anti-ageing effect
Bananas	Potassium, amongst other nutrients	Keeps consistent water levels, maintains heart rhythm
Onions and garlic	Allicin	Beneficial for the heart
Broccoli, cabbage and beans, and other green vegetables	Vitamins A and C, as well as iron, magnesium, calcium, folic acid and fibre	Good for eyes, boosts energy, healthy gums, strengthens immunity and much more
Avocados	Vitamin E	Great for the skin, but quite high in fat so should be eaten in moderation

* Vitamin C is good for healthy gums and bones, boosts immunity and has many other benefits.

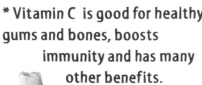

'Fast food'

Convenience foods, which include fast-food takeaways, snacks and ready meals, are becoming increasingly popular.

Everywhere you go

In many countries, food shops are full of convenience food, such as frozen pizzas, burgers, biscuits and crisps. These foods seem to outnumber fresh ingredients like vegetables and meat that people use for cooking. On many high streets we see lots of fast-food restaurants and other convenience food shops.

In the USA alone, the fast food industry is worth $112 billion. ▶

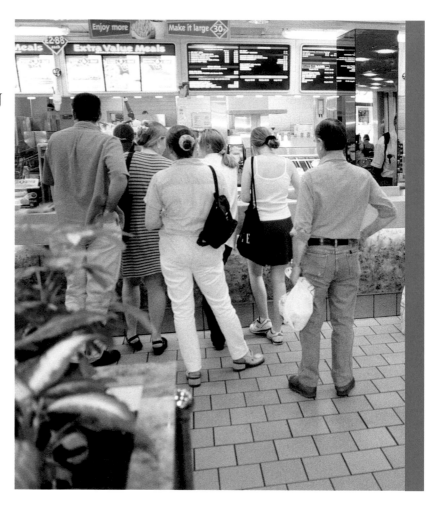

It's your opinion

In the USA, people who have eaten certain convenience foods have sued the people who made them, claiming that the foods are very addictive because of the high levels of fat and sugar in them. They say these foods have made them overweight and they believe such foods should have health warnings on the packets. Do you think they are justified in taking this action?

Convenience foods are usually high in sugar, fat or salt to make them have a longer shelf life and to improve flavour. This means that if we eat them too often they can be bad for our health.

The rise of fast food

People have always enjoyed fatty, sugary foods but there is growing concern in countries like the USA and the UK, and increasingly in newly developing countries, about how much fast food people eat and the impact it is having on health.

Too tempting

There is nothing wrong with enjoying fast foods occasionally, but for many people it is the main part of their diet. One UK survey found that four out of five children aged 4 to 18 regularly ate snack foods such as chips, biscuits and chocolate, but one in five of those asked ate no fruit at all.

Not only are fast foods increasingly popular, but also the size of the portions on offer is bigger. The charity World Cancer Research Fund has found that over the last 20 years, the average hamburger has become over 100 per cent bigger!

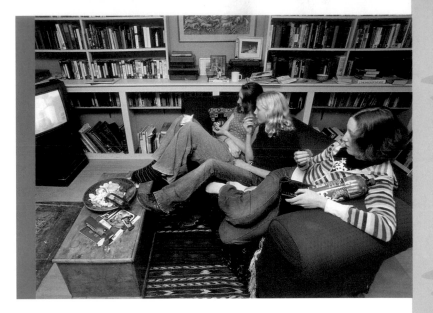

Research has proved that people eat much more snack food in front of the television than they would if they ate a proper meal over a shorter period at the table.

Changes

Some of the world's largest convenience food manufacturers are responding to these concerns. Fast-food giant McDonald's has recently introduced new 'healthy eating' foods, such as salads and wraps into its restaurants.

TV chefs and food writers are trying to teach people that meals cooked from scratch can be just as fast as 'fast foods'. A basic tomato-based sauce with pasta can be made in 15 minutes, half the time it takes to heat a ready meal.

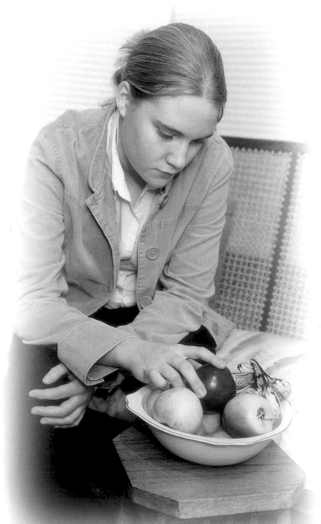

Real fast food! Fruit is the easiest, quickest food to pick up when we are on the go.

It's your experience

'My dad always takes fruit with him to work; he says it is the ultimate fast food – convenient, tasty and healthy – all at the same time!'

Fran, aged 13

What's in your food?

Today most of the food we buy is packaged in some way. This protects the food from getting dirty, makes it easier to handle and also gives food manufacturers a way to say what the food is.

Most food is covered in labelling, partly for advertising and partly to give us information about the food.

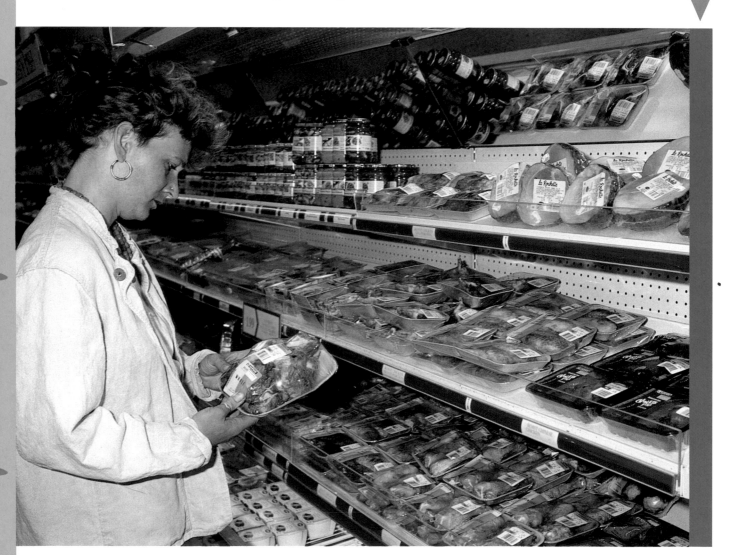

Facts and figures
If you look at food packaging it will tell you the size of the portion you are buying. This is measured in grammes or kilogrammes for dry food and millilitres and litres for liquid food.

Almost all packaged food also have a list of the ingredients. This starts with the ingredient that is used in the highest quantity through to the least-used ingredient. Sometimes percentages are included to show the amount of some or all of the ingredients.

Nutritional information

Many packaged foods have a panel that shows nutritional information about the food. This panel tells us how much of the food is made up from fats, proteins, carbohydrates and vitamins, and also how much energy the food contains. The information usually shows the amount of each nutrient in the food per 100g (grammes), not always the amount in a serving, so you'll have to use your mathematical skills to work out how much is in each portion!

If you look at one of these panels you will see that the levels of nutrients for various foods are very different. Butter, for example, contains a very high amount of fats and almost no carbohydrates or proteins. Bread is high in carbohydrates and fairly low in fats.

All this information helps us to check what is in our food. This may be because we want to eat or avoid certain foods or we need the information to help us build a healthy, balanced diet.

It's your experience

'I went to the supermarket to do the shopping for my mum and dad the other day and it was so confusing. There was so much information on all the packets that I gave up looking in the end and just bought what looked nice.'

Bella, aged 15

Misleading labelling

Sometimes the labelling on food gives extra information. Some labels claim the food is low in fat, high in certain vitamins and minerals, or perhaps high in fibre. They may even claim to be part of a 'healthy eating' range of foods.

This type of labelling can be rather misleading; just because a food is good for you in one way doesn't mean that overall it's healthy. Some breakfast cereals, for example, are very low in fat but are also extremely high in sugar and salt. If you want to eat healthily it's best to ignore these claims and actually check what's in the food yourself.

Nutritional information

Typical values per 100g

Energy	155kJ / 37Kcal
Proteins	1.3g
Carbohydrates	6.8g
(of which sugars)	1.7g
Fats	0.5g
(of which saturates)	0.1g
Fibre	1.4g
Sodium	0.3g

It's your decision

Look at some of the labels on the food in your cupboards at home. Can you tell from the nutritional information what is healthy food and what is not? If the food has labels that say it is healthy, do you agree?

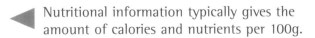

Nutritional information typically gives the amount of calories and nutrients per 100g.

25

Dieting

Being very overweight can be bad for you, and many overweight people try to diet – to lose weight – in order to improve their health. Other people wish to diet because they think it makes them look more attractive.

Diets

If we eat more calories than our bodies use, we will put on weight. If our bodies use more calories than we eat, we will lose weight. On a 'calorie-controlled diet' we only eat a certain amount of food every day, with the aim of losing some weight. When dieting like this people usually avoid eating sugary or fatty foods.

In the short term calorie-controlled diets can be a very successful way of losing weight. There are lots of products that can help people diet in this way, including low-fat and low-sugar meals and snacks.

There are countless other diets that people use to try to lose weight, such as only eating vegetables and raw food or only eating food that is rich in protein.

It's your opinion

'There are no bad foods, just bad diets.' What do you think the nutritionist who wrote this means?

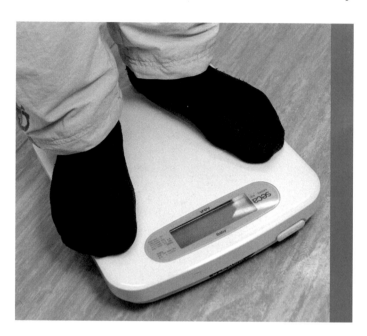
If we want to keep a regular check on our weight, it's best to do it at the same time of the day.

Does dieting work?

Many people find they can lose weight on a diet, but when they finish it they put the weight straight back on. During a diet the body can lose some muscle, which requires more calories to maintain. After the diet we have less muscle – therefore less energy requirements – so have a lower metabolic rate. When we start eating normally again our bodies no longer need the amount of energy being eaten and we put on weight. That is why it is important to exercise during and after dieting.

People who go on a diet sometimes find they think about food all the time, because they know they are not supposed to eat too much. For some people the temptation is too much. They end up eating more than they would have done and then put on extra weight!

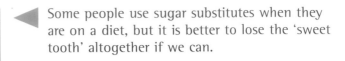

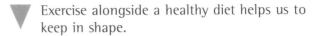
Some people use sugar substitutes when they are on a diet, but it is better to lose the 'sweet tooth' altogether if we can.

Exercise alongside a healthy diet helps us to keep in shape.

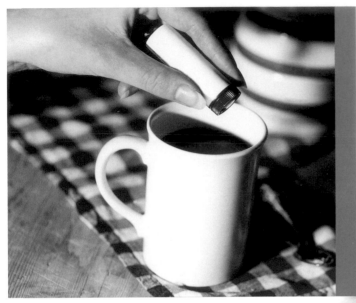

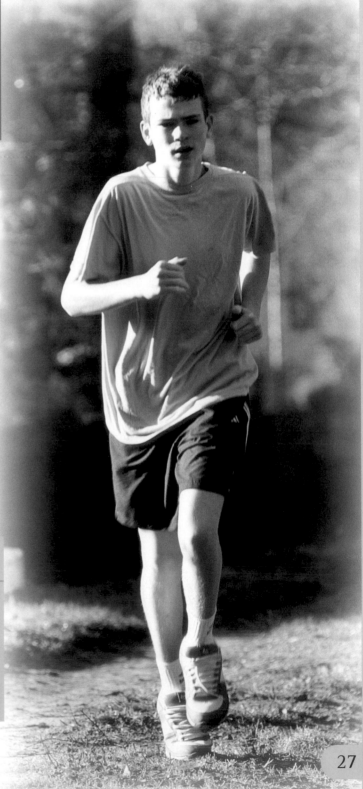

Diets for life

Many people who have lost weight in the long term say that it was nothing to do with going on a diet. They found that making changes in their lives also altered how they feel about food, and helped make it less of a focus.

Leading an active life, including exercising at least three times a week and eating a healthy, balanced diet, including plenty of fruit and vegetables, should help us maintain a healthy body shape. If we are very overweight our doctor can advise us on how to go about losing weight safely.

It's your decision

People usually go on a diet because they want to be healthier or because they think they will look better if they weigh less. If you ever decide to go on a diet, for which reason would it be?

Eating disorders

Eating should be something pleasant, when we can enjoy different foods and perhaps spend time with friends and family. For some people though the whole business of food becomes something of a nightmare.

Anorexia nervosa

If someone has anorexia they become obsessed with losing weight and start eating very little as they are afraid of gaining weight. Anorexics tend to have a distorted view of their own body shape; if someone with anorexia looks at himself or herself in the mirror they may well think that they are fat, when in fact they are underweight and very thin. Doctors think that people become anorexic as a way of showing that they are unhappy.

Health consequences

If anorexia is left untreated, the sufferer will become thinner and thinner. This will eventually have terrible consequences for their health, including irregular heart beat patterns, infertility, weakening bones and growing hair all over the body. In severe cases it can cause death.

Some anorexics grow out of the condition as they get older, but others need hospital treatment and counselling to explore why they have the disease. Anorexia is a serious disease that affects mainly teenage girls. Recently though, younger girls and an increasing number of boys have also been affected by it.

▼ For someone with an eating disorder their weight can be a source of great anguish.

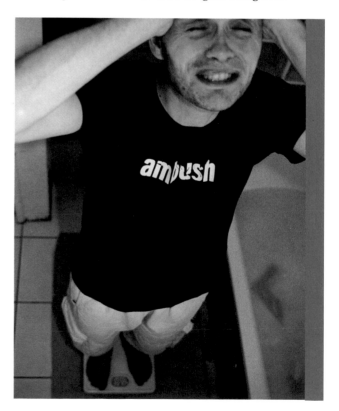

It's your experience

'I was under a lot of pressure at school and I didn't like myself – how I looked and how I acted. What I put in my mouth was something that I could control – and I liked being thin. Eventually I ended up in hospital. One day one of the people I was talking to made me realise that I could die. It's been difficult but I don't want to die so I am getting better gradually.'

Beth, aged 14 (recovering anorexic)

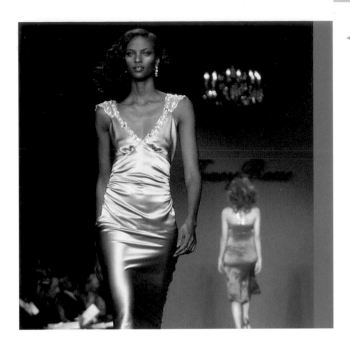

Some people think that stick-thin models make normal-sized people dissatisfied with their weight.

Bulimia nervosa

Bulimia is a condition where sufferers eat large amounts of food, and then vomit. This means that their bodies do not have a chance to absorb the energy from the food and they do not put on any weight.

As with anorexia, doctors believe that people with bulimia are unhappy for some reason. Bulimia is more common than anorexia but it is not as life-threatening. However, excessive vomiting can cause tooth decay, bad breath, and stomach disorders which may have serious long-term health consequences. Sufferers often need counselling and education about healthy eating.

Binge eating

Other eating disorders include bingeing – when a person eats huge amounts of food at one time, and food phobia – where a person refuses to eat certain foods. Phobias are particularly common in small children, but they usually grow out of them.

Bulimia sufferers eat large amounts of food, such as cakes and biscuits, and then throw it up.

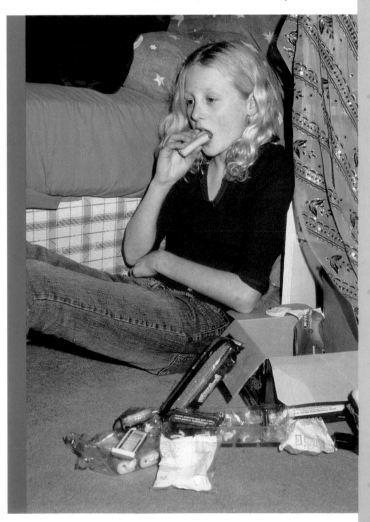

Food allergies

People can be allergic to all sorts of things. Some people get 'hay fever' – a reaction to pollen in the summer months. Others find that being around animals brings them out in a rash. For about one per cent of adults and about four per cent of children, food can cause allergies that can sometimes be very dangerous.

Food allergy

A food allergy occurs when our body reacts in an unusual way to something we have eaten. If we eat a food that we are allergic to, we will start to feel unwell, perhaps getting a headache or a rash on the skin. Some people are so allergic to certain foods that they get a reaction called anaphylactic shock. This can cause sickness and rashes, and sometimes swelling in the throat. In rare cases this can lead to suffocation and even death although it can usually be treated with anti-allergy drugs.

People who know that they are allergic to foods take great care to keep them out of their diet. Peanuts, eggs, shellfish, milk and gluten are the most common foods that cause allergic reactions. Many shops and restaurants now label their food and issue warnings that their produce contains ingredients to which some people may react badly. Scientists do not completely understand why some people react badly to eating particular foods or why allergies are on the increase.

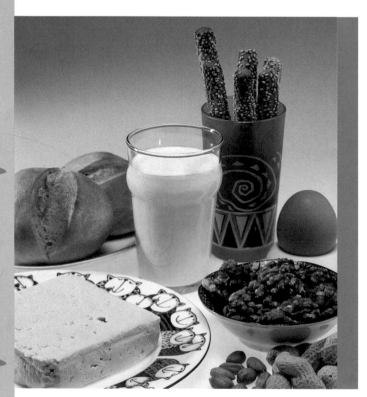

It's your opinion

Many people claim that the food they eat makes them unwell. Do you think food is blamed too often for ill-health?

Dairy foods, bread, eggs and nuts are all foods that can cause allergic reactions in some people.

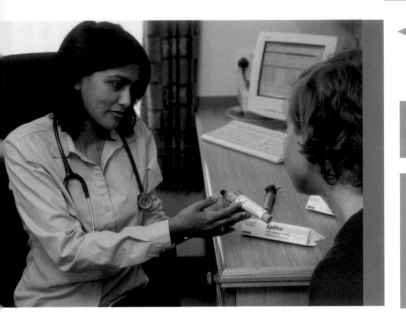

Some allergy sufferers are given epinephrine by their doctors. This is injected during a serious allergic reaction.

It's your experience

'I have coeliac disease and it's a real pain. If I eat anything with wheat in it I get a really upset tummy. You wouldn't believe how much food contains wheat; pasta, bread, pies, cakes, even some sweets!'

Antonio, aged 15

Food intolerance

Food intolerance is much more common than an allergic reaction, affecting about one in five people, but is usually less serious. It is often caused because the sufferer lacks certain enzymes that they need to digest particular foods. A few foods contain strong chemicals that some people find hard to cope with. Coffee, for example, contains a chemical called caffeine that can cause upset stomachs and headaches. Food colourings can affect the behaviour of some people.

Food intolerance is not dangerous, and the best way of coping with it is to simply avoid eating the food that causes the problem. Often people outgrow the intolerance and find that they can eat that food a few months or years later with no problem.

Coeliac disease

People with coeliac disease are intolerant to gluten, the protein found in wheat, rye, oats and barley products. If they eat gluten products they cannot digest their food properly and can become very ill. This is a particularly difficult condition to live with as so much of the food we eat contains wheat. As many as five in every 1,000 people suffer from coeliac disease in countries like the UK, Australia, Canada and the USA.

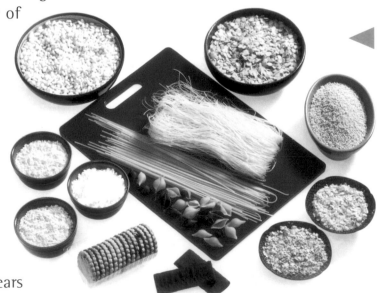

There are many gluten-free substitute products for coeliac sufferers.

Food hygiene

Food hygiene has always been an important part of cooking and eating. Fresh, clean food tastes better than old or dirty food; it is also much safer to eat.

Good food hygiene

You cannot usually tell if food contains bacteria by looking at it but there are simple ways of avoiding food-poisoning:

✓ Meat must be cooked long enough and at the right temperature to make sure any bacteria are killed.

✓ Food should be stored at the right temperature before and after it is cooked. The coldest part of the fridge is the bottom. Storing meat and fish at the bottom also reduces the chance of it dripping down to contaminate other food in the fridge.

✓ Raw food should be stored separately from cooked food.

✓ Shops should always be certain that their food is safe when they sell it.

✓ Anyone who touches food or cooks with it should make sure that they wash their hands thoroughly and that they are not suffering from a stomach upset.

✓ Keep kitchen surfaces clean.

What makes food dangerous?

Tiny bugs, called bacteria, are all around us as well as being in much of the food we eat. Most of these bacteria are completely harmless; indeed some of them are actually good for us. The enzymes used in the digestion process can kill many harmful bacteria.

However, other bacteria, such as salmonella, and E coli and listeria, can be extremely dangerous. Bacteria like to grow in high-protein foods, such as meat and dairy products, and if the conditions are right they can grow very quickly. If we eat food contaminated with dangerous bacteria we may get a very upset stomach. Sometimes people even die from food poisoning.

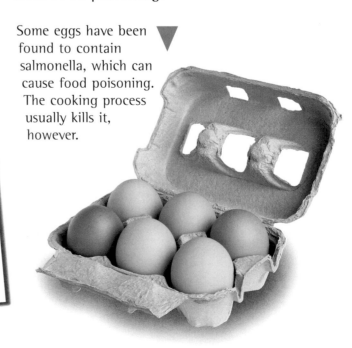

Some eggs have been found to contain salmonella, which can cause food poisoning. The cooking process usually kills it, however.

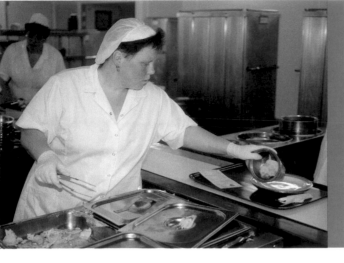

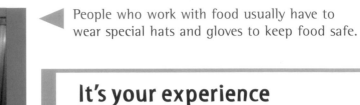

People who work with food usually have to wear special hats and gloves to keep food safe.

How are we protected?

Environmental health inspectors regularly inspect all shops and restaurants that sell food. This ensures that they come up to the right safety standards. If inspectors decide that a shop or restaurant is not safe, it may be closed.

At home there are plenty of ways to keep food safe. Always keep the kitchen very clean and if you want to keep food fresh for longer, you can refrigerate or freeze it.

It's your experience

'I went out with my older brother recently, and we got a take-away from a van. We both got really bad food-poisoning – my brother even had to go to hospital to be re-hydrated. The local council are taking the owner of the van to court now as they say his kitchen fell well below acceptable standards'.

Tom, aged 16

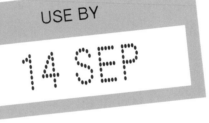

USE BY

14 SEP

Use by dates

If you look at food that has been bought in a shop you will notice that it has a date printed on the packaging. This date shows when the food should be eaten by. 'Best before' dates indicate the time up to when the food will taste fresher. 'Use by' dates show the date after which it is not safe to eat the food.

It's your opinion

Every year many thousands of people suffer food-poisoning from food they have prepared themselves. Many of these cases are due to dirty conditions and food not being stored correctly. Should kitchens in the home have safety inspections to check that they are fit places to prepare food?

Raw and cooked foods should be kept separate in the fridge and well-wrapped.

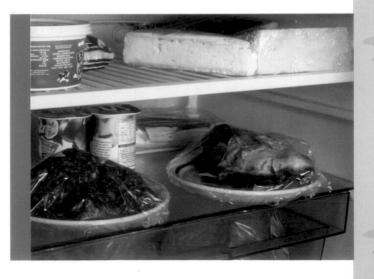

33

Food scares

We all want to know that our food is safe to eat. Sometimes though people disagree as to whether certain foods are dangerous or not.

Additives

Many of the packaged foods we eat contain additives. Additives are used to preserve food, add colour and taste, to make food thicker or to last longer. If you look at the nutritional labelling on different foods you will see that many list E numbers in their ingredients; these are additives.

Some people try to avoid foods that contain E numbers, as they believe they may cause allergic reactions. The flavour enhancer monosodium glutamate, found in many convenience foods, may cause headaches and tightness in the chest.

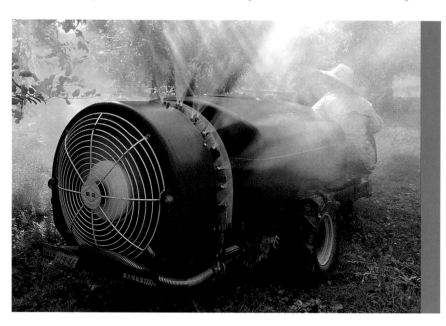

▲ Fruit, vegetables and cereals are sprayed with pesticides on most farms.

Pesticides

Most farmers spray their crops with chemicals called pesticides, which protect them from pests and diseases. They also use drugs, including antibiotics, to keep the animals well. Scientists have shown that some of the chemicals, including organophosphates, are potentially harmful to humans.

Organic food

Some people are worried that pesticides and antibiotics are still in the food when it is sold in the shops. As a consequence there is increasing demand for organic food.

To gain the label 'organic' only natural substances are used to protect and feed the crops and a set period of time has to pass if any drugs have been used on the animals. Organic foods are more expensive than other foods and scientists are a long way from agreeing about the health benefits.

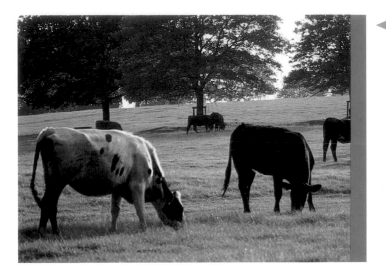

Some people gave up eating beef after BSE in cows was found to be transferable to humans as vCJD.

It's your decision

Over the past few years companies have started to introduce genetically modified, or GM, food. Do you trust the evidence that says this food is completely harmless for humans?

BSE

In the 1980s farmers in the UK noticed that some of their cattle were infected with the disease BSE (Bovine Spongiform Encephalopathy), also known as 'mad cow disease'. The cows probably caught the disease from eating food made from the bodies of diseased animals. BSE affected 178,000 British cattle and resulted in the eventual destruction of 3.7 million animals. British beef has now been declared safe to eat, but the crisis has made some people concerned about eating any beef.

By the mid-1990s scientists realised that people who ate meat from BSE infected cattle could develop the disease vCJD (variant Creutfeldt-Jakob disease); this disease affects the sufferer's brain, and leads to death. No one is sure how many people have vCJD, but more than 100 people have died of the disease worldwide, mostly in the UK. In late 2003 US officials confirmed the USA had its first case of BSE.

Concerns about GM foods have led environmental groups to launch peaceful protests.

GM food

Scientists are now able to identify the genes in crops that are responsible for certain characteristics, for example, resistance to disease. This has led to a revolution in farming – genetically modified, or GM, crops. However some people are concerned about GM. They think that GM crops will adversely affect our health – possibly leading to allergic reactions and increased resistance to antibiotics. At the moment, however, no one knows exactly what the costs and benefits of GM foods are.

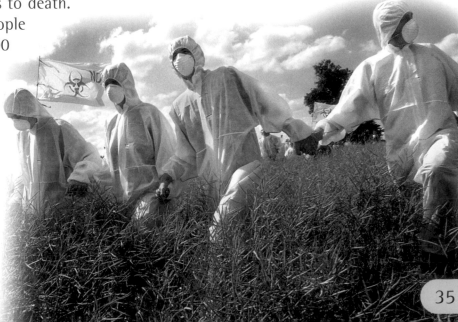

Eating on principle

Some people choose not to eat certain foods because of their beliefs. They may be following religious rules or their own personal belief that it is wrong to kill animals for food. Others simply don't like the taste or texture of meat or fish.

Religion

Many religions forbid the eating of certain foods, although members of those religions sometimes vary on how seriously they take these restrictions. In Islam, all meat is halal, (slaughtered according to special rules). Eating pork is also forbidden, as is drinking alcoholic drinks.

In Judaism people do not eat pork or shellfish and all their food is kosher. One important aspect of kosher food is that meat and dairy products are stored, prepared and eaten separately.

In the Hindu religion cows are considered sacred and are not killed or eaten. Many Hindus are vegetarian, believing it is wrong to kill animals for food. Some other religions also have different dietary restrictions.

Protection

All of these dietary rules are very old. As well as being important parts of the religion for spiritual reasons, they may well have helped protect their followers in a more practical way. Food-poisoning and contamination was hard to control in the age before refrigeration and modern cleaning methods, and many of these food laws would have helped keep people safe from diarrhoea and sickness. This is still true for many people in the poorer countries of the world.

It's your decision

Do you have principles relating to food? Is there anything you wouldn't eat because you think it would be wrong?

A kosher kitchen has two sinks: one for dairy products, and one for meat.

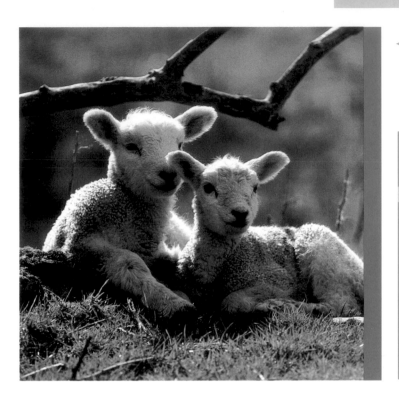

◀ Although some vegetarians like meat, they refuse to eat it because they believe it's cruel to animals.

It's your opinion

▶ Do you think the vegetarian diet is necessarily healthier than other diets? Vegetarians may avoid potentially dangerous fats in red meat but they may well eat them in cheese or butter. How easy do you think it is to eat a balanced vegetarian diet?

Vegetarianism

Vegetarians do not eat meat and fish, while strict vegetarians, known as vegans, also avoid dairy products and eggs. Vegetarianism has become very popular in countries like the US, Australia and the UK. About one in twenty of the UK population is vegetarian and across Europe over 11 million people don't eat meat.

Some vegetarians believe that their diet is a much healthier than one that includes meat, because it is high in fibre and low in the saturated fats found in some meat. Others argue that a vegetarian diet is not natural and that our bodies were designed to eat meat. They suggest that a vegetarian diet is low in protein and lacks vital vitamins, such as B12, which are only found in animal products. Most nutritionists however agree that a balanced vegetarian diet can be extremely healthy as long as pulses are used as well as dairy products for protein.

Some vegetarians use tofu, which is full of protein, as a substitute for meat in their cooking. ▶

Food and the media

Adverts are everywhere; on television, in newspapers and magazines, even on the sides of buses. Many of these advertise food, and some are aimed specifically at children.

 TV advertising sometimes has an almost hypnotic effect on young children.

Advertisements

In some countries, like Sweden and Norway, it is illegal to advertise junk food to children. Their governments believe that children are too young to make up their own minds about what to buy.

In most other countries food companies are free to advertise to young people and many of the advertisements on children's television and in magazines 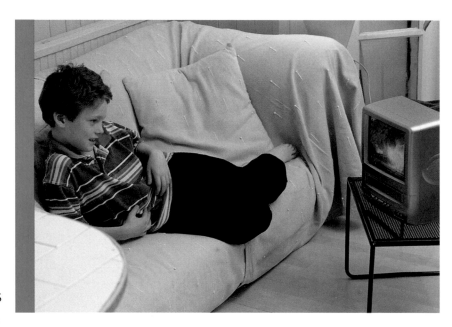 promote their products. Most food that is advertised, including soft drinks, crisps and chocolate, is high in fats, sugar and salt, which can cause health problems if consumed in excess.

Childhood obesity rates are highest in countries where there is the least TV regulation – USA, Australia and the UK.

Advertisers deliberately market to children as they believe children influence what the whole family eats.

It's your opinion

Famous sports stars often appear in adverts for soft drinks and snack food. What sort of example do you think they are setting?

It's your experience

'Every time a new children's film comes out, my little brother goes mad for all the stuff that goes with it. Last time the fast food restaurants were doing a promotion that went with the film. He pestered my mum so much that we ended up going practically every other day.'

Jill, aged 15

Many foods are marketed at young children. Often these foods are full of sugar or salt.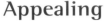

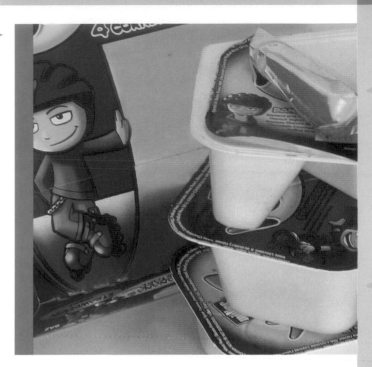

Appealing

Even if we do not see adverts for food, once we are in the shops we can't fail to notice the foods that are promoted by popular children's characters. Some foods feature cartoon characters on their labels which encourage very young children to pester their parents for the food. Other foods use images of the latest films and pop personalities to encourage older children to buy them.

Healthy-eating drives

Television characters can of course have a postive effect on eating habits. Popeye the sailor, who acquires super-strength by eating spinach, had a huge impact on children's eating habits after first appearing in an American cartoon strip in the 1920s. In the UK, 'The Food Dudes', a cartoon series that features characters that fight to save the world from 'General Junk' and his army of vegetable-hating 'junk punks'. Children who watched the cartoon are found to eat more fruit and vegetables.

Backlash

Because of criticism some food and drink companies have agreed to stop marketing their products to children. Heinz has said it will not target any advertising for its products solely at pre-school children, though it will continue to use pictures of TV characters on its packaging. In the USA several states have banned the sale of sweets and fizzy drinks in schools.

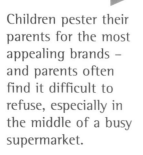

Children pester their parents for the most appealing brands – and parents often find it difficult to refuse, especially in the middle of a busy supermarket.

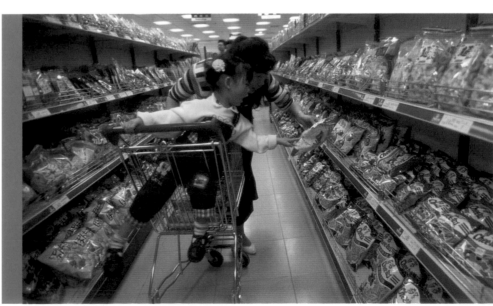

Food and you

You may not have thought too deeply about food before; after all eating is such a basic need for each and every one of us. When you do think about food though you realise that there are all sorts of issues to consider.

In France, buying food from markets is a way of life because the food is very fresh and cheap.

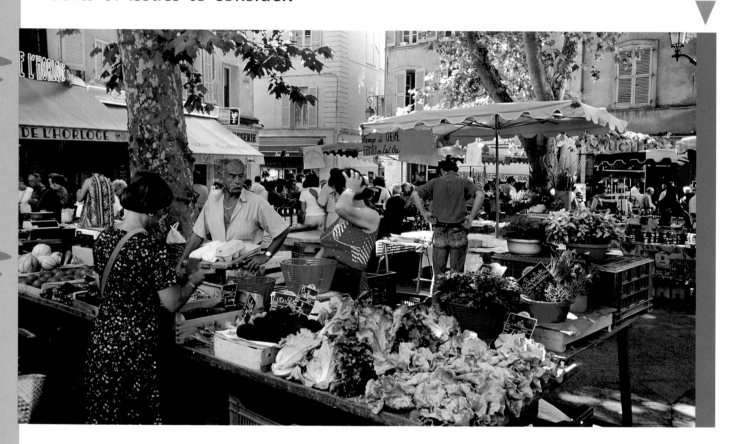

It's your opinion

How much of the responsibility for healthy eating can lie with teenagers? Should school meal providers and parents think more about what they cook? What about snacking? Where does the responsibility lie there?

Health and convenience

It may seem that we have to make a choice between eating the foods that we really enjoy and eating healthily. If we eat convenience foods all the time we may put our health at risk, but there is nothing wrong with enjoying these things as part of a balanced diet. Many people say that they enjoy simple foods like salads and vegetables much more than processed foods.

Stages of your life

What you eat will be likely to change throughout your life. Fashions for different foods will change and things that are currently not available will be sold in the shops. Your dietary needs will also change; as a teenager you may well need huge amounts of energy to help you grow and keep you active. As you get older you will probably find you need to eat less.

For women, becoming pregnant or breastfeeding a baby may also lead to a change in their diet.

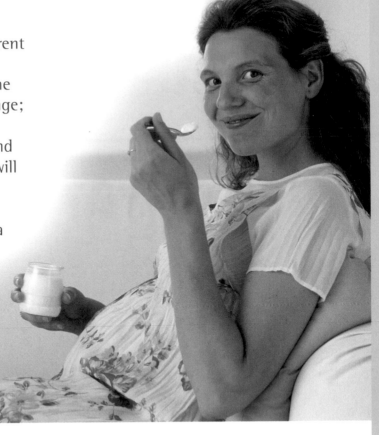

Pregnant women have to be careful about what they eat. ▶

Taking control

You may well find that cooking your own food becomes more important to you as you get older. There are many popular programmes on television and numerous books showing how you can cook all sorts of delicious meals. If you do start cooking, you will soon realise that there is no end to the choice of healthy and delicious food that you can eat. Cooking your own food is also a lot cheaper. Whatever you eat in the future, remember that eating can and should be one of life's most enjoyable experiences.

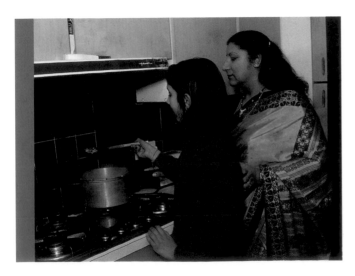

It's your experience

▶ 'My dad started to teach me to cook last year. Now I always watch the cookery shows on Saturday morning and cook my family a meal on Sunday to try out some recipes I've seen.'

Toby, aged 15

◀ Cooking can be a social and enjoyable experience.

Glossary

Bacteria a group of living things, which cannot be seen with the naked eye. Some bacteria can cause diseases

Balanced diet a diet that contains all the food we need for a healthy body, in the right proportions

Calorie a measure of the energy value of food. We need to eat a certain amount of calories each day depending on our size and level of activity

Carbohydrates substances, found in foods such as bread and pasta, which are the body's main source of energy

Cholesterol a substance, found in animal fats, tissues and blood, which can cause heart disease if there is too much in the body

Diabetes an illness where a person has too much sugar in their blood because the body does not produce enough insulin

Diet the type and amount of food a person eats each day

E coli a bacteria that can cause serious food-poisoning

Fats substances that supply the body with energy and help to insulate it

Fibre a substance found in plant foods that helps the body's digestion

Heart disease when fatty substances build up inside the coronary arteries, which supply the heart with blood

High blood-pressure when blood pushes against the walls of our arteries too hard

Infertility inability to produce a child

Insulin a substance that regulates the amount of sugar in the blood

Junk food food that is low in nutritional value, which is eaten as well as, or instead of, a proper meal

Listeria a bacteria that can cause serious food-poisoning

Mineral one of over 20 substances, including iron and calcium, needed in a person's diet to maintain good health

Nutrient a substance found in food, such as carbohydrates, proteins, fats, minerals or vitamins, needed to work the body properly

Osteoporosis when bones become weaker due to lack of calcium

Processed food food that has been altered from its original state by a special treatment, for example, to stop it decaying or to make it taste different

Proteins substances used by the body for growth and repair

Salmonella a bacteria that can cause serious food-poisoning

Stroke a potentially fatal bleeding in the brain

Soya bean an Asian bean that can be used to make flour, margarine, oil and milk

Vitamin one of over 13 substances, including vitamins C and D, needed in small amounts in a person's diet

Further information

Websites:
www.bbc.co.uk/food/healthyeating/
Offers guides to healthy eating to show how a good diet can leave you with more energy and vitality.

www.exhibits.pacsci.org/nutrition
Activities to do with food and eating.

www.nutritionaustralia.org
A website featuring information about nutritional values and food labels.

www.readthesigns.org
Lists organisations that specialise in problems such as eating disorders.

UK organisations:
Food Standards Agency
Protects the public's health and consumer interests in relation to food, including healthy eating and food labelling.

Aviation House, 125 Kingsway
London WC2B 6NH
Telephone: 020 7276 8000
Website: www.foodstandards.gov.uk

The Soil Association
A leading campaigning and certification organisation for organic food and farming.

Bristol House, 40-56 Victoria Street
Bristol, BS1 6BY
Telephone: 0117 929 0661
Email: info@soilassociation.org
Website: www.soilassociation.org

The British Nutrition Foundation
Promotes nutritional health with information on the latest scientific studies.

High Holborn House
52-54 High Holborn
London WC1V 6RQ
Telephone: 020 7404 6504
Email: postbox@nutrition.org.uk
Website: www.nutrition.org.uk

Australia and New Zealand organisations:
Food Standards Australia New Zealand
(formerly ANZFA)
Protects health and safety by maintaining a safe food supply.

PO Box 7186, Canberra BC ACT 2610, Australia
Telephone: +61 2 6271 2222
Email: info@foodstandards.gov.au
Website: www.foodstandards.gov.au

PO Box 10559, The Terrace, Wellington 6036, New Zealand
Telephone: +64 4 473 9942
Email: info@foodstandards.govt.nz

Index

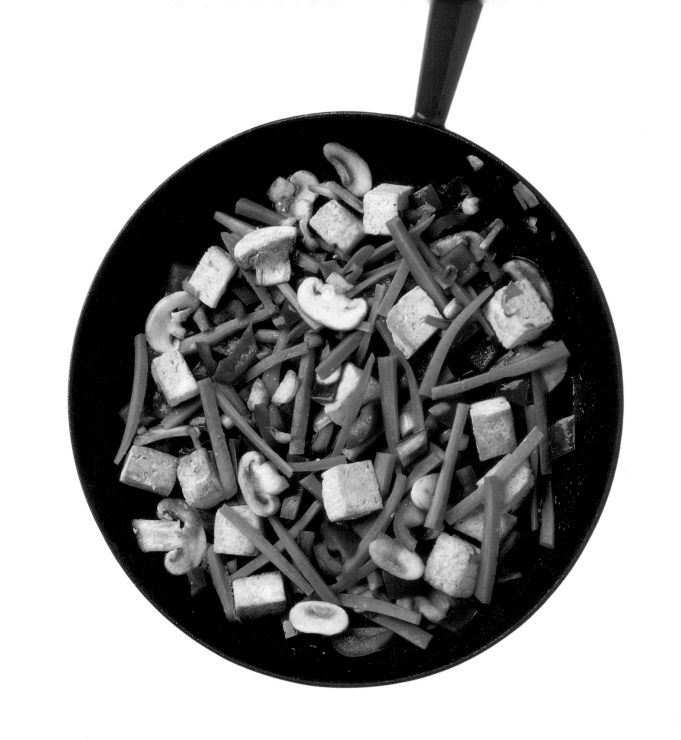